KIRTAN ANGELS

By

Krishna Devi

AuthorHouse™
1663 Liberty Drive, Suite 200
Bloomington, IN 47403
www.authorhouse.com
Phone: 1-800-839-8640

First published by AuthorHouse 05/06/2008

ISBN: 9-781-4343-7025-9 (sc)

Printed in the United States of America
Bloomington, Indiana

This book is printed on acid-free paper.

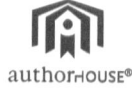

authorHOUSE®

Dedication

This book is dedicated to all the Kirtan Bhaktas who give their lives selflessly through chanting and sound vibrations, which brings peace and   love to all beings - they are " Kirtan Angels".

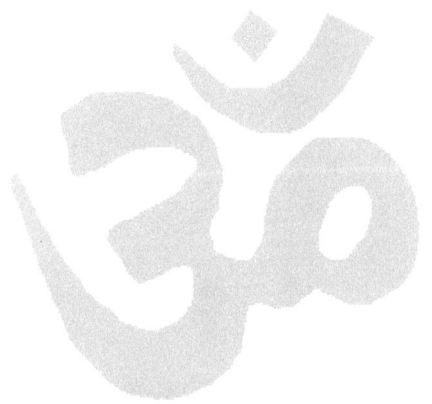

**OM DYAUH SHANTIR, ANTARIKSHAM SHANTIH,
PRTHIVI SHANTIR, APAH SHANTIR,
OSHADHAYAH SHANTIH, VANASPATAYAH SHANTIR,
VISHVE DEVAH SHANTIR, BRAHMA SHANTIH,
SARVAM SHANTIH, SHANTIR EVA SHANTIH,
SA MA SHANTIR EDHI.
OM SHANTIH, SHANTIH, SHANTIH.**

OM. MAY THE HEAVENS BE IN PEACE AND HARMONY.
MAY THE SPACE BE WITHOUT POLLUTION.
MAY OUR MOTHER EARTH BE PEACEFUL AND FREE FROM
ALL POLLUTION.
MAY ALL THE WATERS BE PEACEFUL AND FREE FROM ALL
POLLUTION.
MAY ALL MEDICINAL HERBS AND PLANTS BE IN THEIR
NATURAL STATE.
MAY THE WHOLE VEGETABLE KINGDOM, INCLUDING
TREES AND FOREST, BE HEALTHY AND FREE FROM
POLLUTION.
MAY ALL THE ELEMENTS AND ALL COSMIC FORCES BE IN
PEACE AND HARMONY.
MAY ALL OF EXISTENCE BE IN PEACE AND HARMONY.
MAY EVERYTHING, IN AND OUT, BE PEACEFUL AND FREE
FROM POLLUTION!
AND MAY PEACE ITSELF BE REAL PEACE.
AND LAST BUT NOT LEAST, MAY THAT NATURAL PEACE,
HARMONY AND UNITY MANIFEST THROUGH US!
MAY THERE BE PEACE, PEACE, PEACE - PHYSICALLY,
MENTALLY, AND SPIRITUALLY.

— Translated by Shri Brahmananda Sarasvati —

Acknowledgements

First thank you to my Guru Shri Brahmananda Sarasvati of Ananda Ashram, Monroe, NY for all his Teachings and Love.

Acharya Roop Verma for his Foreword writing, Teachings and Music.

Edited by Shawnte Salabert.

Cover Picture - Bhavani Lee.

Cover Photo by Juren David.

Advice and Research - Gene Loeb.

Text Layout and Cover Design - Dinesha Barber.

Contents

Foreword

A SPIRITUAL PATH TO HIGHER CONSCIOUSNESS
By
Acharya Roop Verma, M. Mus. Sangitalankar.

Krishna Devi has been a dear friend and a spiritual sister walking the hard and delicate path of self-discovery. I first met her in 1975 at the Summer Convocation of the Yoga Society of New York at Watson Homestead in upstate New York. It was the grace of Guru Shri Brahmananda Sarasvati that brought many of us to walk the path of Yoga, which seemed fun in the beginning. But it didn't take long to realize the nature of this journey and the razor-like awareness it demanded.

I was still living and teaching in Ottawa, Canada, but Ananda Ashram, the Guru and all spiritual friends became more and more inseparable from me as the time passed. And then I made one of the most important decisions of my life: to move to the ashram in the summer of 1977.

It was the start of a new chapter for me, and Krishna was my foremost friend to help and support during the times I was most vulnerable spiritually to distractions. I came from a spiritually minded yogic family and thought I had a good background, but Krishna's compelling and selfless devotion to Guru, God and the path became so very inspiring to actually help me look at my own inner path. It was the time when Guruji Shri Brahmananda was intensely teaching the Yoga Sutras of Patanjali and the Devi Mahatmyam and 'Self Analysis'. It became clear to me very soon that it was a 'once in a lifetime' opportunity to study and grow under the direct guidance of Guruji.

I thank Krishna Devi and am honored to have been asked to write the 'Preface' for her book about Kirtan. Her Kirtan chanting, although simple, to this day has a resonance and a soul quality, a rare glow, which promotes that inner inquiry. As I look back, my own spiritual journey began from Kirtan when I was still in middle school in India. So it feels right in my heart to say what I have known and experienced through this extraordinary and yet simple form of devotional music, which truly has a transforming power.

Although dynamic at times but deeply sublime at its root, Kirtan is the most ancient devotional musical form, precursor of the Classical Indian Musical system.

It is the very heart of our spiritual life. It means singing, chanting and praising different aspects of God as our true essence. Kirtan uses tools common to all forms of world music, namely tones and rhythms, to enhance the experience of musical resonance – to intensify it. This intensification is stress free as it does not violate the laws of nature's integral harmony that governs all creation.

Kirtan is a simple and most powerful form of chanting to access the field of Tattvas, the elements, and eventually transcend them, leading human awareness towards inner silence and meditation. Almost always, a few lines of a mantra or poetry are included in the Kirtan to give a meaning for the satisfaction of the wandering logical mind, which seeks to feed on new forms and thoughts constantly.

The goal of Nada Yoga is that the logical thinking consciousness be merged into "sound consciousness" by repetition of a Mantra, Kirtan or Bhajan and other yogic means which, at their peak climax experience, become a pure resonance of sound (Nada).

In this journey of pure love and devotion, the Kirtan becomes a powerful step to lead us into a state of vacuum, so to speak, where there are no walls or barriers or mountains to cross. You are catapulted into that space of highest awareness spontaneously where meditation is no more an effort. And, therefore, meditation and Kirtan have been practiced since the beginning of the first human urges to know his/her source; 'who am I and why I am here'. Kirtan answers that inner inquiry and helps the wandering mind to focus and observe itself through the sense of hearing, whereby it can become one pointed – a pre requisite to meditation (Dhyana).

THE MAGIC FOLLOWS!

Thus, Kirtan is rightfully regarded as a unique blend of Bhakti Yoga and Nada Yoga and does not concern itself with other complex rules of classical musicality. Its solitary goal is to re-unite our split awareness into its source.

Patanjali speaks about the 'extraordinary sense perception' in Yoga Sutras, Chapter I, verse 35.

Since ancient times, musical instruments used for Kirtan have also been simple; namely an Ektara which later evolved into Tamboura. Later on, many other forms of cymbals, bells, tambourines and drums of various sizes and shapes were added. However, the most important and powerful instrument is the human voice - the inner calling of the individual soul - as it comes to re-align itself in resonance and synchronicity with others. One does not have to be, or pretend to be, a performer at all but only to chant with open heart and soul.

Kirtan, considered as a branch of Nada Yoga, is a path of exploring consciousness through sacred music, which originated in the ancient Vedic times. It is one of the most direct ways to access the field of Self where the distinction between Self and non-self, our desires and their substitutes, can be identified. There is an untouched 'space' within each one of us, which does not know fear, sickness and suffering of any kind. It is always in a joyful state of perfection. Through Kirtan, you can enter the state of meditation and enhance the quality of your life.

Meditation is now recognized the world over due to its enormous benefits physically, psychologically and spiritually. It revives and restores our equilibrium that begins to disintegrate due to harsh, rough and crude vibrations we all experience almost every day. Although meditation is a purely scientific and non-religious yogic process, it can be easily adapted to any form of religious rituals/practices. Singing a Kirtan in a group unites our minds on one 'single focus' and can be a powerful prayer.

With all my love and blessings,

Acharya Roop Verma, M. Mus. Sangitalankar.

Oneonta, New York, November 13, 2007

" GURU DEVA BRAHMANANDA

SHARANAM MAMA OM"

Introduction

I was inspired to write this book about Kirtan because my life is dedicated to god realization through Bhakti yoga and Kirtan chanting. I want to share with you this divine healing and the joy of chanting.

I see that the practice of Kirtan is growing more and more here in the West. The world is not an easy place to inhabit right now, but Kirtan brings healing and peace to your mind. Unlike studying and reading philosophy—which, in time, may or may not bring healing and happiness—chanting devotional Kirtan is a direct and immediate method of feeling happiness and spiritual oneness.

At that time, one experiences the opening of the heart.

My spiritual knowledge and practice comes largely from my Guru, Shri Brahmananda Sarasvati (Ramamurti S. Mishra), who I studied with at Ananda Ashram in Monroe, NY. This is a place where Kirtan, chanting, mantra, Sanskrit, music, and meditation are always in full bloom. Although I grew up learning different kinds of music and songs, the ashram is the place where I discovered and learned about Kirtan and chanting—mostly from my Guru, but also from the late Ramesh Lahiri.

I received a lot of musical training in my younger age. I grew up with Gypsy music, especially that of my grandfather. He was my very first teacher in music and as a little girl, I danced to his violin and cello, the sounds of his playing bringing happiness to me.

In the beginning I didn't realize why I enjoyed so much to chant god's name. However, gypsies original came from India.

Their music comes with feeling directly from the heart, so there is a deep connection for me in both forms.

At Ananda Ashram's Blue Sky Theater, the best Kirtanists come and go. The theater is full of magnetic energy all of the time; sometimes it feels as if ancient India has come to us with Kirtan, chanting, classical music, sitar, tabla, and countless artists sharing the sound of divine energy.

The meditation room is where thousands of programs have been conducted and it is where I chant my Kirtan every Sunday. This is a holy place, so divine with burning candles, fragrant incense, and a room where mantras or Kirtan have been—and still are—chanted every morning and night, with homa and fire ceremonies conducted to increase world peace and healing.

The meditation room is also where Swami Bhakti Vedanta, on his first visit from India, chanted the Maha-Mantra. The energy is very powerful in this room; our Guruji used to meditate and chant there at least twice daily.

All of these mantras and Sanskrit are still practiced every day with different teachers, including Bharati (disciple of Shri Brahmananda Sarasvati) and Dr. Sharma (world-renowned Sanskrit professor from India). Joan Suval is also teaching here every weekend. Many other scholars come and go, sharing their wisdom. Also Acharya Roop Verma is teaching music, Nada Yoga and giving heavenly concerts.

I've been watching the growth of Kirtan chanting for a long time, and I don't always like what I see because sometimes, the chanters forget the real meaning of Kirtan. This book is written for all of the chanters and bhaktas, so that we may keep the real meaning and essence of this healing art intact. The world needs more godly presence and one place in which it can be found is in this ancient healing art of Kirtan.

I am not from India. I was born in Europe, but since coming to Ananda Ashram, I have experienced a great deal of training in sound vibration, Sanskrit, healing, meditation, and the understanding of worship and the universal meaning of symbols. I want to share my experience with you.

Can you imagine a place with no pain or sorrow, where the sun shines equally on everyone? A place where one can experience the highest happiness—feeling god-like, feeling free, walking without fear, smiling and seeing that oneness in each other's eyes, living with an open heart and peaceful mind, feeling a love like that which is usually only dreamt about? A place where birds always sing happily, where one can breathe fresh air perfumed with the fragrance of roses, drink crystal-clear water, dance in the rain, and almost touch the blue sky and all of its rainbows?

The description above is our earthly right. Great yogis experience all of these things I've described through meditation and Samadhi, but to bring about world peace, each and every person has to purify their mind and enter into meditation to experience our oneness. Right now, this seems like a dream, but some Gurus say that after Kali Yuga, a beautiful world will once again exist, where we will all live in the highest happiness. Everyone will be god-like and see only one love in each other's eyes.

So, for this purpose, we should keep chanting and purifying our mind. We should trust and have faith in god, so that we can fly above the clouds where the sun always shines. We should all keep dreaming and chanting god's name.

Death is just like changing your clothes. On the stage, actors wear different costumes and change behind the stage, much like we all "dress up" for the different phases of our lives. God protects us and he keeps a veil in our mind, so that we don't remember our past lives until we are ready to remove the veil. Gurus know our past lives and they know how far we have come with our spirituality. They know and experience that the real existence of consciousness contains an awareness, and that its nature is pure bliss.

Chapter 1

WHAT IS KIRTAN?

Kirtan is the devotional chanting of sacred sounds and god's names. If this is your path, you can realize god through Kirtan chanting alone. It is the easiest way to attain the feeling of oneness and is the best medicine for the mind. Group chanting and prayer is the heart of yoga; it is a healing energy and an integral part of Bhakti Yoga, which incorporates giving oneself to the divine.

Kirtan belongs to Pratyahara, the fifth element of the eight limbs of yoga in which you draw the mind inward and withdraw the energy from the senses for a higher purpose. Kirtan connects the inner and outer self and awakens the stillness and peace within. Repetition of the sacred names and syllables purifies and brings the mind into the present. It does not matter which names you choose to chant, as long as you have devotion in your heart.

The combining of words, melody, and rhythm in a spiritual way can be very powerful. Chanting is a prayer and repetition provides the building power to intensify one's own prayer. Kirtan is not for sentiment and emotion, but rather for the inner purpose of bringing the heart to a place of higher consciousness. Chanting dissolves the thinking mind.

After chanting, listen to the sound of "Aum" (Om) emanating from the head and throughout the entire body. Music is the vibration of "Aum", which is ultimately what we are. Chanting is praying, talking to god; after you listen to "Aum", god is chanting and talking to you.

If you lead Kirtan, you do not need to be a great musician, but pronunciation and respect for the godly language, Sanskrit, is very important. You must pay attention to whether the vowel is short or long, if the consonants are dental, palatal or labial, and other important language details. Each letter and syllable is an energy point, like acupuncture for the brain. When properly used, it awakens the kundalini energy and one begins to feel the inner pulsation; this energy body brings you to your god and to your higher self. This is the place where sorrow and pain disappear. This is our healing journey.

We are currently in Kali Yuga, approaching its end. Through Kirtan, we are inviting the next yuga, Satya Yuga or "the golden age." By chanting, we are inviting god and we become the bridge between Kali Yuga and Satya Yuga. In Kali Yuga, the only way to live is by chanting god's names; it takes away the pain from the world. The proper technique of chanting brings energy, enlightenment, healing, and peace to the world.

If you chant Kirtan, it doesn't mean that you become Indian or Hindu—although we have a lot of respect for this beautiful, ancient, and godly land. You don't need to change your religion—god's vibration belongs to all. All of this beautiful knowledge, mantras and Kirtan, comes from the East and we are the West. By practicing and bringing all of this inward, we become the true East-meets-West, the true unity of yoga.

Our Guruji loved the American disciples; he would not let anybody touch his feet. In India, you bow down and touch the master's feet—he did not want that; he just wanted to teach and help all of his students. He did not want us to become Indian, but simply to become godly.

We worship god in a form of a person because it's very hard to worship just the blue sky, the energy in nothingness, or the unknown force.

Kirtan chanting makes you fly and enter into ecstasy. By clapping, dancing, and drumming the rhythms of the music with harmonium and bells, everyone becomes one pulsation and one breath, feeling oneness and timelessness. Dance and sing with your beloved god and take him into your heart. This is the energy and love that transforms you and the world; then you will see only love and god in each other's eyes. The chanter disappears into ecstasy and the blue sky. The mantras protect the mind from thinking. Mantras are blessings.

Kirtan is chanting and repeating god's names in a melodic, musical way.

Japa is repeating god's names on mala beads.

Bhajan is singing stories of love and expression about god.

The Kirtanist should know about Bhakti yoga, learn Sanskrit pronunciation, and serve the world. Nowadays, you can listen to Kirtan on radio stations. We can listen to god's name anytime, but Kirtan should be kept sacred and special in the original and most powerful form. We have to adopt a proper mental attitude and feeling (bhava) to chant and keep god's names as simple as possible, with a deep respect for the divine.

Sometimes Ananda Ashram's Blue Sky Theater is so charged with the heavenly sounds of musical vibration that the elements react. One can actually move the elements through sound vibration.

These concerts are always dedicated to world peace and healing. There are two kinds of healing; one type occurs through reading and studying non-dualistic philosophy. With this type, seeds are planted in the mind, and these seeds may grow and ripen, with that person eventually experiencing healing. The second type is direct and immediate healing. Instant healing is felt right away through many experiences—by sitting with an enlightened being, by chanting Kirtan from the heart with humility and devotion, by hearing divine music, mantra, through dancing or watching devotional dance.

GAN GAN GANAPATI

NAMO NAMASTE

Prayer to Ganesha to remove all obstacles.

OM SHRIM NAMAH

This Laksmi mantra brings prosperity.

OM NAMO NARAYANI

Salutations to the Divine Mother.

SATYAM SHIVAM SUNDARAM

Feel the truth, tranquility and beauty.

OM SHANTIH, SHANTIH, SHANTIH

Peace.

Chapter 2

SANSKRIT LANGUAGE

Sanskrit language is the mother of all languages. It is a cosmic language that can transform your mind and it has the power to unite the whole world through chanting. It can raise our minds and hearts from lower to higher.

There are fifty letters in the Sanskrit alphabet. Fourteen of these are vowels, including long, short, and diphthong forms. The consonants have five categories—gutturals, palatals, cerebrals, dentals, labials—and they are hard or soft, with semi-vowels and sibilants mixed in. There are different conjugations and case endings, as well as sandhi rules that you must follow. Sandhi occurs when a word followed by another word undergoes changes. There are also variations of past tense, active and passive voice, and levels of more advanced study, including Panini grammar.

With our Guruji, we chanted every day for hours and hours, until our thinking mind was dissolved and we felt only pulsation. While sitting with the guru and chanting, your mind undergoes various changes and transformations. Our Guruji was a medical doctor, but he knew that outer medicine does not heal the mind; the medicine that he used was Sanskrit chanting and grammar. When you chant in the presence of a great guru, his physical being also elevates your mind.

BHARATI DEVI

She is a very dedicated disciple of Shri Brahmananda Sarasvati.
Her chanting and speech are inspired by Goddess Sarasvati herself.
She leads programs and teaches Sanskrit at Ananda Ashram.

SARASVATIM NAMASYAMI CETANAM HRIDI

SANSTHITAM,

KANTHA-STHAM PADMA-YONIM TVAM HRIN-KARAM

SUPRIYAM SADA.

" We need a divine language to unite our hearts and minds for world peace. Sanskrit vibrates deep layers of the psyche through pranic vibration. All mantras are based on the pure science of sound vibration, Sanskrit is quantum healing for body and mind, and the language of the heart and unity,the language of integration."

— Shri Brahmananda Sarasvati —

Chapter 3

BRANCHES OF YOGA AND THEIR MEANING

Yoga means "union", and there are many branches that explore various forms of union:

Hatha yoga—physical posture and asana

Raja yoga—mental work and study

Karma yoga—service and work

Bhakti yoga—devotion to yoga in your heart

Tantra yoga—ritual

Mantra yoga—energy-based sound

Kirtan chanters use both Bhakti yoga and Mantra yoga. Everyone can chant and praise god's names, but if you lead Kirtan, you must study and learn about Bhakti yoga, mantra, Sanskrit, and meditation.

Bhakti yoga is the yoga of love and devotion. Bhakti comes from the root bhaj—to worship. The devotee wants to be alone with god and divine grace comes from devotion. Before you chant, silently offer yourself to the universe as a divine instrument.

There are nine forms of Bhakti:

Shravana — hearing

Kirtana — chanting

Smarana — remembering

Padasevana — service

Archana — worship

Vandana — prayer

Dasya — servant of god

Sakhya — friend of god

Atmanivedana — surrender

Single-minded bhakti means sacrificing all other supports and relying on god alone.

—Bhakti Sutra, sutra 10

Whenever his glory is invoked—Kirtan—god manifests himself soon and makes the devotee experience him.

—Bhakti Sutra, sutra 80

Bhakti gives peace, bliss, and divine ecstasy.

Raja yoga focuses on the intellect and the mind. This is when we study the Yoga Sutras and Upanishads to develop our mind; while studying, we also chant the verses. In the Yoga Sutras, the eight steps of yoga are:

Yama – The laws of the external world.

Niyama – The laws of the internal world.

Asana – Physical body postures.

Pranayama – Breath control.

Pratyahara – Withdrawal of the senses.

Dharana – Single focus.

Dhyana – Continuity of the flow of energy.

Samadhi – Complete absorbtion with the Divine.

Hatha Yoga incorporates a diverse array of styles, for example:

Ashtanga vinyasa and Jivamukti Yoga — power yoga

Dharma Yoga — Created by Dharma Mittra

Ananda Yoga — more gentle (founded by Swami Kriyananda)

Anusara Yoga — flowing with grace (founded by John Friend)

Bikram Yoga — hot yoga (founded by Bishu Ghosh)

Integral Yoga — pranayama, meditation, and posture (founded by Swami Satchidananda)

Iyengar Yoga — alignment of posture, including the use of props like blocks and belts

Kali Ray Tri Yoga — create a flow with asana, using breath and mudra

Kripalu Yoga — work with individual flexibility and strength

Kundalini Yoga — breath, asana, movement (founded by Yogi Bhajan)

Sivananda Yoga — set structure (founded by Vishnu Devananda)

Swaroopa Yoga — opening the spine (founded by Rama Berch)

Vini Yoga — flow of breath and movement of spine (founded by Krishnamacharya)

No one form of yoga is better than the other; it is your personal choice to choose the style that feels right for you.

Chapter 4

HISTORY OF KIRTAN

There are many different ways of chanting. These include Gregorian chants and Buddhist chants in monasteries, Christian chants in churches, Kabbalah Kirtan, Lila Kirtan (Lila means "the play" of Shri Krishna and it is sung directly to him), Sikhism Kirtan (one of the pillars of Sikhism—singing of the sacred hymns in classical rag style), and Gurbani Kirtan (daily chanted prayers).

Overall, Hindu or Sanskrit chanting is the most popular form. Variations of chanting or singing exist in every religion, but Sanskrit chanting is a godly language. It creates a completely different feeling, a direct communication to universal energy and pulsation, and enters your heart right away.

In ancient times, words and music were used to attain altered states of mind, with music being used to develop the mind, develop the spirit, and heal the emotions. When you combine bhava (deep feeling) with Kirtan or mantra, the energy intensifies. The expression of supreme devotion and love is the heart of Bhakti Yoga.

Many mantras are difficult to translate fully into English. If you chant a mantra thinking of its meaning, you will not go beyond the mind, because meaning belongs to the mind. When we chant the mantra hundreds of times, the mind becomes *rasa* (emotion) and that rasa becomes *soma*, the pure ecstasy of joy.

NARADA MUNI

Narada Muni was a great devotee of Krishna (Vishnu). His name means "the one who gives knowledge to mankind and guides them on the right path," and he has spread the path of devotion.

Narada sang praising god. It is said that he was the inventor of the first musical instrument, the veena, a stringed instrument made from a gourd. He was loved by all, and as such, he appears in all three yugas. His aim is to convert people to bhakti, believing that in Kali Yuga the chanting of the lord's name will bring greater reward than by simply doing sacrifices alone.

OM NAMO BHAGAVATE VASUDEVAYA

HARI HARI BOL, KRISHNA KRISHNA BOL

MUKUNDA MADHAVA KESHAVA BOL

RADHE RADHE BOL, GOKULA BOL

MUKUNDA MADHAVA KESHAVA BO

Narada came to many writers like Vyasa and Valmiki to share his belief that the path of devotion is the best. The best known of his works is the Narada Bhakti Sutra.

CHAITANYA MAHAPRABHU

Chaitanya Mahaprabhu was a Vaisnava monk of Bhakti yoga in the 15th century. He worshipped Radha and Krishna and popularized the chanting of the Hare Krishna mantra. His teaching is about the pure love of Radha and Krishna and he was totally absorbed by this. Chaitanya started the very first "SanKirtana," congregational devotional singing.

SHRI KRISHNA CHAITANYA, PRABHU NITYANANDA

HARE KRISHNA HARE RAM, RADHE GOVINDA

JAY RADHE KRISHNA, JAY RADHE KRISHNA

JAYA JAYA NANDALAL, GIRI DHARA GOPALA

HE GOVINDA HE GOPALA, HE DAYALAL

A.C. BHAKTIVEDANTA SWAMI PRABHUPADA

On the order of his guru, Srila Bhaktisiddhanta Saraswati Thakura, A.C. Bhaktivedanta Swami Prabhupada brought the teaching of Shri Chaitanya from India, spreading it around the Western world. He began in New York and circled the world fourteen times, fostering awareness of the Hare Krishna movement. He also created the International Society for Krishna Consciousness (ISKCON) for followers of Bhakti Yoga.

HARE KRISHNA, HARE KRISHNA

KRISHNA KRISHNA, HARE HARE

HARE RAMA, HARE RAMA

RAMA RAMA, HARE HARE

JAYA RADHA-MADHAVA, JAYA KUNJA-VIHA

JAYA GOPI-JANA-VALLABHA JAYA GIRI-VARA-DHARI

JAYA YASODA-NANDANA JAYA BRAJA-JANA-

RANJANA

JAYA YAMUNA-TIRA-VANA-CARI

MIRA BAI

Mira Bai expressed love and devotion in poetic form in the 15th century and even now, her words still touch people's hearts. She believed that she was Lalita, one of Krishna's gopis, and she sang and danced in a trance, just to please her lord.

I looked for the dark-one,

I found his image in my heart,

I stood in his court,

My life in his hands,

Only his medicine healed.

— Mira Bai—

Chapter 5

THE DIVINE PLAYS

RAMAYANA is a dance drama involving the mythological life of Shri Rama. It is a divine map to enlightenment. You will find that every character in the Ramayana is a symbol for the mind; it is one's internal journey. Pancavati, the city of five gates, represents our five senses. This Ramayana is our inner story and journey through meditation, wherein all of the characters represent your inner self.

Ravana, the ten-headed demon, represents the ego and Shri Rama represents your divine soul. Through many obstacles, Rama kills Ravana, and at the end, he becomes the king of Ayodhya (our physical body), which represents the divine taking over your being.

We all have to walk the same road towards enlightenment. The difference is that some people get there faster than others—this is the journey that we all take if we meditate. All of the Ramayana verses can be chanted and the vibration of this drama can be felt. The gurus say that the more you watch the show or chant the Ramayana, the more you can eliminate different karmas.

Shri Hanuman, the monkey god, represents cosmic energy and prana. Chanting the Hanuman Chalisa is especially known to reduce the sorrows in the world.

Valmiki, the writer of Ramayana, was a very bad man whose mantra was "Mara," which means, "to kill." He repeated it like a japa and through repetition, "Mara" became "Rama." Through this sound vibration and the power of Rama's name, Valmiki became a divine man and he wrote the Ramayana.

SITA RAM, SITA RAM, SITA RAM, JAYA SITA RAM

DEVI MAHATMYAM is also known as CHANDI MAHATMYAM and DURGA SAPTASHATI. There are 700 verses celebrating the triumph of the divine over the forces of evil. The divine mother is not just a poetic verse; we actually receive help and simply chanting these Sanskrit verses reduces our pain. They are usually chanted on specific days in the spring and in the fall.

JAYANTI MANGALA KALI BHADRA KALI KAPALINI

DURGA SHIVA KSHAMA DHATRI

SVAHA SVADHA NAMO 'STU TE

—Salutation to all forms of Kali-

OM MATA KALI, SHRI MATA KALI

OM MATA KALI SHRI DURGE

OM MATA, SHRI MATA

OM SHRI MATA, DURGA MA

OM DURGE, SHRI DURGE

OM SHRI DURGE, JAGADAMBA

ATMA BODHA (Self Knowledge)
Composed by Shankaracharya

These are verses about self-knowledge—they refer to the
eternal question "Who am I?" They are used for purifying
our mind and heart through self-discipline and also for those
who have an intense desire to experience the one energy as
their own self.

TAPOBHIH KSHINA-PAPANAM

SHANTANAM VITA-RAGINAM

MUMUKSHUNAM APEKHSHYO 'YAM

ATMA BODHO VIDHIYATE.

This Self Knowledge, "Who am I" Atma Bodha, is
composed for those who have purified their hearts by tapah
(self discipline), whose hearts abound in tranquility, whose
minds are free from the pairs of opposites (such as personal
love and hatred), and who have intense desire to experience
Brahman as their own Self.

Atma Bodha (Self knowledge)
Composed by Shankaracharya
Translated by Shri Brahmananda Sarasvati

YOGA SUTRAS
Composed by Patanjali

Yoga Sutras of Patanjali is the most used and famous book and is an essential tool for all yogis. It describes the limbs of yoga, cosmic psychology, the absolute "I-Am," the process for transforming the individual mind to the universal mind, and explains supernatural powers.

YOGASH CHITTA-VRITTI-NIRODHA.

Yoga (Union) is the cessation of the thinking mind

SA PURVESHAM API GURUH

KALENA ANAVACCHEDAT.

Being beyond time and space, God is the guru of even the ancients, the guru of all gurus and the master of all masters. He is always within the heart as the sad-guru.

TAJ-JAPAS TAD-ARTHA-BHAVANAM.

One should chant OM vocally and mentally and should focus one's flame of attention on the inner OM, the inner cosmic music, anahata nadam, which is the music of the inner voice, the inner silence.

— Translated by Shri Brahmananda Saraswati —

BHAGAVAD GITA

The Bhagavad Gita, or "song of god," is a conversation between Krishna and Arjuna that occurs on a battlefield, representing our own battlefield of life. Krishna is the speaker in this Gita (as Bhagawan), communicating with Arjuna, the devoted seeker. The verses are written in poetic forms and are easily and melodically chanted:

MAYYEVA MANA ADHATSVA MAYI BUDDHIM

NIVESHAYA

NIVASISHYASI MAYYEVA ATA URDHVAM NA

SAMSHAYAH

Fix your mind on me alone, let your thoughts dwell in me,

you will hereafter live in me alone, of this there is no doubt.

— Bhagavad Gita, Bhakti Yoga, verse 8 —

Chapter 6

CHANTING THE DIFFERENT NAMES OF GOD

To do anything in this world, or if you want to chant, you have to know and feel "I-Am," which means "absolute god." There are different gods' names used for the different aspects of our true nature.

The most important gods' names to chant are: Ganesha, Rama, Sita, Narayana, Laxmi, Shiva, Shakti, Parvati, Durga, Kali, Krishna, Govinda, Gopala, Radha, Buddha, Jesus, Allah, Kali, Bhavani...and many, many others.

GANESHA

VAKRATUNDA MAHAKAYA

SURYA KOTI SAMA PRABHA

NIRVIGHNAM KURU ME DEVA

SARVA KARYESHU SARVADA

Oh Lord Ganesha of large body and curved trunk

With the brilliance of a million suns

Make all my work free of obstacles always.

Ganesha is the son of Shiva and he is the remover of obstacles and giver of success.

He is the ruler of the first (red) chakra. He has two wives: Riddhi, who represents material wealth, and Siddhi, who represents spiritual wealth. Above all else, Ganesha is the destroyer of all obstacles.

GANESHA SHARANAM, SHARANAM GANESHA

GANESHA SHARANAM, SHARANAM GANESHA

Take refuge in Ganesha

SHRI GANESHA SHRI GANESHA PAHI MAM

SHRI GANESHA SHRI GANESHA RAKSHA MAM

Shri Ganesha protect me.

KRISHNA

Krishna is an incarnation of Vishnu in Dvapara Yuga. His skin is a dark blue-black and his crown is the peacock feather. He is both magnetic attraction and the blue sky; he represents the living pulsation of Om. Krishna conquers the demons, and is the lover of gopis. In addition, he is sometimes known by other names, including Gopal (a boy playing with the cows), Govinda (he pleases and controls the cows, or senses), Hari (lord of nature), and Murali (one who holds the flute).

All the bhaktas love Krishna, especially if one is a romantic. Many times, you see Krishna playing the flute, but the flute is not really there. This invisible flute is the sound of Om, which charms both the gopis and Radha. Om pleases the senses and the mind. When you hear this divine sound, meditation occurs and through the sound, you unite with your beloved Krishna.

Radha is the extension of Krishna. Her love to Krishna demonstrates the highest ecstasy of love and the act of feeling it is called mahabhava—the ultimate depth of feeling of love. Radha Krishna is like the sun and the sun's rays— there is no difference. This has a very special meaning in Samkhya yoga, when the individual mind is totally absorbed in god through magnetic energy and bliss.

One of Radha's names is Krishnamaya, which means "the one who sees Krishna both inside and outside." Her name is also Mother Hara, which, in the vocative case, becomes Hare. The deeper meaning of Hare Krishna translates to Radha- Krishna. To reach Krishna, you have to go through Radha.

GOPALA GOPALA, DEVAKI NANDANA GOPALA

GOVINDA JAYA JAYA, GOPALA JAYA JAYA

RADHA RAMANA HARI, GOVINDA JAYA JAYA

Victory to Krishna (Govinda)

OM BHAGAVAN SHRI BHAGAVAN

ANANDA BHAGAVAN, SHRI KRISHNA BHAGAVAN

JAPA RADHA KRISHNA, GOPALA KRISHNA

KRISHNA KRISHNA, SHRI RADHE

BHAJA RADHA KRISHNA, GOPALA KRISHNA

KRISHNA KRISHNA, SHRI RADHE

GOVINDA BOLO HARI, GOPALA BOLO

RADHA RAMANA HARI, GOVINDA BOLO!

SHRI RAMA

Rama is a warrior and he kills the demon Ravana (our ego) and is the incarnation of Vishnu in Treta Yuga. Rama represents the cosmic soul, his brother Laksman represents the individual soul and his wife Sita represents the divine mind, wisdom, and intelligence. The Ramayana is our inner story and journey through meditation.

RAM RAM BHAJA MANA,HARE HARE RAM

SHRI RAM JAYA RAM, JAYA SITA RAM

SITA RAM, SITA RAM, SITA RAM, JAYA SITA RAM.

Victory to Sita and Ram

RAGHU PATI RAGHAVA RAJA RAM

PATITA PAVANA SITA RAM

SITA RAM JAYA SITA RAM

SITA RAM JAYA SITA RAM

HANUMAN

Hanuman, the monkey god, is a main character in the Ramayana; there is no Hanuman without Rama. Hanuman is well loved in Bhakti yoga and Kirtan; he takes away all sorrows and misery. His father is Vayu, the air element, and he taught Hanuman pranayama and subsequently, Hanuman created the Surya Namaskar for dedication to his guru Surya, the sun.

We chant Hanuman Chalisa to remove some of the suffering from the world. Hanuman's mystical meaning is cosmic pulsation and cosmic energy. When we chant, our body fills up with energy and prana, and then we feel the pulsation. By feeling this magnetic energy, our sorrows and pain disappear; Hanuman then becomes Anuman—molecules and atoms. Here, he carries you directly to Rama.

JAYA HANUMAN.

Victory to Hanuman

SHRI HANUMATE NAMAH

JAYA HANUMANA JNANA GUNA SAGARA

JAYA KAPISA TIHUN LOKA UJAGARA

RAMA DUTA ATULITA BALA DHAMA

ANJANI PUTRA PAVANA-SUTA NAMA

KALI

Kali is the mother of the universe, our real mother protecting us in life and death. Her sword is ever ready to cut our ego, so that we can feel ourselves as bliss. She remains always there, watching over us, as we are her children. By crying out and chanting her name, Kali rushes to protect you—you are her child and you can see her in your mind. In your meditation, she is the power of all mantras and Kirtan.

Kali wears on her neck the fifty-one letters of the Sanskrit alphabet, each representing different energies. When you chant with the power of the Shakti, kundalini energy arises and Kali appears. With her ominous sound of hum, all demons disappear—you could be in the middle of war, in the worst situation with nowhere to turn, and at that time, she is there for you. If you go inside yourself, into the emptiness of your mind, and call out her name, she will rush to you with a sword to protect you.

Kali has many names: Durga, Ambika, Bhavani, Amba

KALI DURGE NAMO NAMAH.

Salutation to Kali - Durga.

AMBA BHAVANI JAYA JAYA AMBA.

OM MA KALI MA SADA GURU SHRI MATA

PARA SHAKTI OM MA KALI

SADA GURU SHRI MATA

SARA LA KALI

Sara La Kali is the goddess of the Gypsies and this is the only saint that they worship. In May, she is celebrated in the South of France. She is the goddess of creation, healer of sickness and death, and they all chant her name:

Vive Sara la Kali

They all come under the black night

Under the distant stars

The one who dares to get lost

Queen of Romanies let me lose myself,

let me lose myself,

I am moved, I am moved to roam

To touch my roots to dance,

To fly back to my own home

Don't be afraid of darkness

She'll embrace you

Just listen to her gypsy cry

Eyes pouring into rain

As she enchants me, thousands of miles away

She enchants me

— Queen of Romanies, by Bhavani Lee —

DURGA

AMBA PARAMESHVARI, AKHILANDESHVARI

ADI PARA SHAKTI, PALAYA MAM.

OM AIM HRIM KLIM, CHAMUNDAYAI VICCHE OM.

OM NAMO NARAYANI

DURGAYAI DURGA PARAYAI

SARAYAI SARVA KARINYAI

KHYATYAI TATHAIVA KRISHNAYAI

DHUMRAYAI SATATAM NAMAH

Salutation always to Durga who takes one accross
in difficulties, who is essence, who is the author of
everything, who is knowledge of discrimination
and who is blue-black as also smoke like in complexion.

— Devi Mahatmyam chapter 15 verse12 —

SHIVA

There are three divine aspects of life, represented by three gods:

Brahma is the creator.

Vishnu is the preserver.

Shiva is the destroyer of the world.

Shiva is the god of yogis; he is pure consciousness. As Nataraj, the dancer, Shiva represents destruction and creation, birth and death. As Trayambaka Deva, he grants boons. As Satyam Shivam Sundaram, he is truth, peace, and beauty.

OM NAMAH SHIVAYA

Salutation to Shiva

OM TRYAMBAKAM YAJAMAHE SUGANDHIM PUSHTI

VARDHANAM

URVARUKAM IVA BANDHANAN MRITYOR MUKSHIYA

MAMRITAT.

Oh, omniscient Divinity we adore you. Oh, Lord full of excellent fragrance,
you are the nourisher, the sustainer of all life.
As the ripe cucumber is gently released from the vine
thus liberate us from death and grant us nectar of immortality.

NATARAJA NATARAJA

NARTANA SUNDARA NATARAJA

SHIVA RAJA SHIVA RAJA

SHIVA KAMI PRIYA SHIVA RAJA

CHIDAMBARESHA NATARAJA

PARTI PURISHVARA NATARAJA

KASHI VISHVESHVARA

UMA MAHESHVARA

SADA SHIVA SHAMBHO

SADA SHIVA

NAMAH PARVATI PATAYE HARA HARA

HARA HARA SHANKARA MAHA DEVA

OM HARA OM HARA MAHA DEVA

OM SHIVA OM SHIVA SADA SHIVA

SADA SHIVA MAHA DEVA

MAHA DEVA SADA SHIVA

JESUS

Jesus and all of his stories are well loved. In churches, they worship and chant his name. Jesus tells us to find heaven inside of our own hearts, and to be loving towards all.

Our Father who art in heaven,

Hallowed be thy name, thy kingdom come, thy will be done

On earth as it is in heaven. Give us this day our daily bread,

And forgive us our trespasses as we forgive those who trespass against us.

Lead us not into temptation and deliver us from evil.

For thine are the kingdom, and the power, and the glory, forever and ever.

Amen

SURYA THE SUN GOD

The sun has a physical and spiritual form and it exists as the visible form of god that one can see every day, often symbolizing light and life. In Egypt, the sun god Ra was worshipped; he was the glorious king of the gods. The pyramids were built based on the idea of sunrays. Without the sun, the earth would be a dark and cold place to live. Surya is the living god that everyone can see.

As the chief solar deity, his arms are gold and his chariot is pulled across the sky with seven horses, representing our seven chakras, or energy centers in the body. The Gayatri Mantra is associated with the sun. Millions of people chant and give respect to the sun at sunrise or sunset. The sun gives energy and light. Sun meditations are very powerful, especially at sunrise because we can stare at Surya, the sun, when his color is red—this is the only time you can look directly at him. Chant about him and lose yourself in the love of this visible god.

The Spiritual Light that is hidden within the sun is the most excellent light. It shines through the hearts of all living creatures in the form of consciousness. The Spiritual Light that is shining within the physical sun also shines within the heart of every being. This Light is more brilliant than fire or a comet. The Light that is shining in the heart of all jivas (individuals) in the form of consciousness and awareness is also shining through the universe in the form of Surya's rays.

GAYATRI MANTRA

BHUR BHUVAH SVAH, TAT SAVITUR VARENYAM

BHARGO DEVASYA DHIMAHI,

DHIYO YO NAH PRACHODAYAT OM.

Almighty Supreme Sun impel us with your
divine brilliance so we may attain a noble
understanding of reality.

Most of the gods come in pairs. Some gurus say that we
have a mother and father god; that is the way in which both
ourselves and the universe were created.

Brahma and Sarasvati

Vishnu and Lakshmi,

Sita and Rama,

Radha and Krishna

Shiva and Shakti

NAMAMI SHANKARA BHAVANI SHANKARA

UMA MAHESHVARA TAVA SHARANAM

NAMO NAMO SHIVA MAHADEVA

OMKARESHVARA TAVA SHARANAM

OM SHIVA OM SHIVA PARA PARA SHIVA

OMKARESHVARA TAVA SHARANAM

BUDDHA

The Buddha who is the founder of the Buddhist religion is called Buddha Shakyamuni "Shakya" is the name of the royal family into which he was born, and "Muni" means "Able One." Buddha Skakyamuni was born as a royal prince in 624 BC in a place called Lumbini, which was originally in northern India but is now part of Nepal. His mother's name was Queen Mayadevi and his father's name was King Shuddhodana.

OM MANI PADME HUM

"The Jewel in the Lotus"

Tibetan Buddhists believe that saying the mantra (prayer), **Om Mani Padme Hum**, out loud or silently to oneself, invokes the powerful benevolent attention and blessings of Chenrezig, the embodiment of compassion.

BUDDHAM SHARANAM GACCHAMI

ISHAM SHARANAM GACCHAMI

SANGHAM SHARANAM GACCHAMI

DHARMAM SHARANAM GACCHAMI

Chapter 7

MODERN KIRTANISTS – ANGELS OF PEACE

The practice of modern Kirtan includes repeating god's names, with the addition of Western music, using major or minor chords. Sometimes, words are chanted in English, guitar and other Western instruments are used, and the style becomes more folksy, jazzy, or electric.

The following are descriptions of the real pioneers who brought the chanting of god's names to the West.

RAMESH LAHIRI

Ramesh Lahiri was one of my teachers. His voice was so beautiful and soulful; he sang from his heart. Ramesh was from Kolkata (Calcutta), India and he sang Kirtans and bhajans at Ananda Ashram for ten years, before leaving his body. His most mystical chants were about Kali.

JAYA DURGE, JAYA DURGE, JAYA DURGE,

JAY JAY MA

KALI KAPALINI MA, JAYA JAGAD AMBE MA

JAGAD UDDHARINI MA, JAGAD UDDHARINI MA

YOGANANDA

Yogananda created a new kind of chanting, establishing an East-West method. This type of chanting includes the repetition of meaningful phrases, rather than the divine names, becoming more like a personal affirmation. His disciple Kriyananda said, "Music in our time has become increasingly disconnected, nervous, violent and out of touch with the source that used to nourish it and give it meaning. If this trend continues—and it shows no sign of reversing itself—the cost to our society will be enormous, even explosive."

Some of Yogananda's chants are:

I am the bubble, make me the sea.

So do thou, my lord. Thou and I, never apart,

Wave of the sea dissolve in the sea,

I am the bubble, make me the sea.

Why, o mind wanderest thou?

Go in thine inner home.

KRISHNA DAS

Krishna Das is the father of Kirtan in the West, the New Messenger who popularized Kirtan in this part of the world. He is one of the most beloved Kirtanists.

Krishna Das studied with his guru Neem Karoli Baba in India, practicing Bhakti yoga, immersing himself in worship and love for his guru. Now, he leads programs and Kirtan all over the world. What I enjoy about Krishna Das is his friendliness to all. He is very natural and doesn't prefer to wear the orange clothes of sadhus, but he speaks of god and prays like a true holy man.

SHAMBHO SHANKARA NAMAH SHIVAYA

GIRIJA SHANKARA NAMAH SHIVAYA

HARA HARA MAHA DEVA SHAMBHO

KASHI VISHVANATHA GANGE

BOM BOM MAHA DEVA SHAMBHO

KASHI VISHVANATHA GANGE

JAYA JAGAD AMBE

SITA RADHE

KALI DURGE

NAMO NAMAH

"If we know anything about a path at all,

It's only because of the great ones that have gone before us.

Out of their love and kindness, they have left some footprints for us to follow.

So, in the same way that they wish for us,

We wish that all beings everywhere, including ourselves, be safe, be happy,

Have good health, and enough to eat.

And may we all live at ease of heart with whatever comes to us in life."

— Kirtan closing prayer by Krishna Das —

SHYAMDAS

Shyamdas is a devotional singer, translator, author, and storyteller. He brings Vedic literature and Bhakti yoga to life in the West. He combines ecstatic Kirtan with beautiful stories of Radha and Krishna, and spiritual teachings from India. He is also a devotee of Neem Karoli Baba.
He blends songs, kirtan, dynamic stories and teaching of the path of devotion A recognized presenter both in the West and in India, he has written and translated more than 20 books on the Yoga of Devotion.
He has studied classical Dhrupada music and divides his time between the U.S. and India.

MAHA RANI KI JAY, RADHA RANI KI JAY

VARSANI VALIKI JAY JAY JAY!

GOVINDA HARE, GOPALA HARE

HEY PRABHU DINA, DAYALA HARE

BHAGAVANDAS

Bhagavan Das, is a teacher, performer, counter-cultural icon, and lover of god. He lived in India for years as a sadhu and his guru is the great Neem Karoli Baba. Bhagavan Das tours constantly, chanting god's name and giving workshops.

The path to enlightenment is not a group trip, it's between you and god.

— From Its Here Now (Are You?) by BHAGAVANDAS —

RAGHUPATI RAGHAVA RAJA RAM,

PATITA PAVANA SITA RAM,

SITA RAM SITA RAM,

BHAJ PYARE TU SITA RAM,

ISHWARA ALLAH TERE NAM,

SABKO SANMATI DE BHAGAVAN.

Translation:

Lord Rama, Chief of the house of Raghu,
Uplifters of those who have fallen, Sita and Rama,
Beloved, praise Sita and Rama,
God or Allah is your name,
Lord, bless everyone with wisdom.

65

JAI UTTAL

The sound of Jai Uttal is truly East-meets-West and world fusion. Coincidentally, his guru is also Neem Karoli Baba. He also learned music and chanting with the street singers (Bauls) and received classical music training early in his life. In 2002, he was nominated for a Grammy Award for Best New Age Album.

 'World music is music from everywhere, music that creates bridges, music that unites hearts and cultures, music that brings peace.'

— Jai Uttal —

RADHA RAMANA HARI BOL, RADHA RAMANA HARI BOL

RADHE RADHE RADHE RADHE BOL, RADHE RADHE RADHE RADHE BOL

RADHA RAMANA HARI BOL.

SWAMI MA CHETAN JYOTI

Swami Ma Chetan Jyoti is a great Kirtan singer and swami. She has an ashram in India called the Shri Krishna Kripa Ashram. Her Guru is Shri Swami Chandra Swami.

Swami Ma Chetan Jyoti is known as "The Queen of Kirtan." Her soulful voice cries out god's names as she chants with harmonium and drums. She visits the United States and Europe once a year. She is the only saint who visits the leper community in India and always brings them their favorite treat, tea.

You are the air I breathe, Shri Ram.

— Swami Ma Chetan Jyoti —

AYODHYA RAJA SHRI RAM

DASHARATHA NANDA SHRI RAM

PATITA PAVANA JANAKI VALLABHA

SITA MOHANA RAM

DEEPAK KUMAR

Deepak has one of the most beautiful voices. Born in Rajasthan India, Deepak lives in the U.S., and tours internationally. He is a classically trained singer,performing many styles of Indian music, including Bhajan, Ghazal, Thumri, Dadra and Kirtan. He expresses so many feelings through his voice. He also teaches vocal music in the classical tradtion.

RAMA RAMA, JAY SHRI RAM

HARE HARE HARE HARE KRISHNA HARE

KRISHNA HARE, KRISHNA HARE, KRISHNA HARE,

KRISHNA HARE

There are many more chanters in the West, including Wah, Ragani, Suzan Green, Manorama, Kamaniya, Durgadas, Milk Baba, and Gandharva. They all are angels of peace.

Chapter 8

TECHNIQUES FOR KIRTAN

First, with our hearts in deep gratitude, to the universe for this amazing blessing of life, we chant using proper Sanskrit pronunciation and a humble, devotional feeling (bhava). This is like cooking a healthy meal that gently nourishes our body. After chanting, through silent feeling, meditating on the vibrations created in every cell of the body and throughout the atmosphere, we nourish our mind, body, and spirit.

The best instruments to use are harmonium, ektar, and guitar, accompanied by drum, tabla, mridanga, and bells. Sometimes violin, cello, or flute enhances the Kirtan.

Before you chant in public, you should have some knowledge of proper Sanskrit pronunciation. This is most important, although even the best Kirtanist doesn't have perfectly correct pronunciation, even in some of the important, daily mantras.

Search for a Guru or teacher and learn about meditation and music. Study Narada Bhakti Sutra and learn that the very first thing is to worship god. Establish your relationship with him—there is an all-loving god and you can find him in your own center.

Always start and end by chanting Om (Aum). The first Kirtan is usually in praise of Ganesha; afterwards, you can sing about different gods. Between each chant, we meditate and the sound still flows in the silence. Each chant should last ten to twenty minutes, and an entire Kirtan session will last between 1 ½ to 2 hours, even all night like Kirtan Party.

The rhythm becomes progressively faster and that gives power and Shakti; freedom to dance is important. Combine feeling (bhava) with the chant and at the end, use mantras for world peace and healing. Then chant Om (Aum) three times and lead everyone to meditation for a few minutes.

The light of the room makes a big difference in the feeling. I prefer a dark room with an assortment of candles, pink or rose-colored soft light, and a picture of your guru or your deity in view—in that way, you feel more comfortable and it becomes just you and your god.

When you are in the spiritual world, you may or may not make much money from chanting. This is your service and healing to the world—and to yourself.

Grace happens from god when you are ready. Unexpected events will happen in your favor and then you enter into a magical world. You receive love in life if you love god in your heart.

ACHYUTAM KESHAVAM RAMA NARAYANAM

KRISHNA DAMODARAM VASUDEVAM HARIM

SHR DHARAM MADHAVAM GOPIKA VALLABHAM

JANAKI NAYAKAM RAMACHANDRAM BHAJE.

Chapter 9

THE GURU AND THE ASHRAM

There is nothing higher or greater in life than learning and studying with a Guru, especially if you live in the ashram and give service. It is a beautiful, peaceful surrender—you experience the sunset and sunrise with holy chanting and sun meditations, walk barefoot on the wet grass, feel the pulsation of energy, feel so free that you could almost fly, and are nourished with the purest vegetarian food. These blessings feel like they will never end.

The Guru knows how to bring you to your highest state of kundalini energy. Later, you have to do this on your own, learning the secrets of yoga from the Atma Bodha andYoga Sutras, purifying your mind through chanting (especially in Sanskrit) and learning music, dance, and meditation so that this showering of blessings may come to you. Then you start the discovering of awareness and learn witnessing of the mind through meditation. You enter into the world of kundalini energy, where everything becomes very magical.

The Guru shows you reality, universal truth, and godly manifestation, sometimes silently, without words. The ashram feels like home and you feel so safe and protected that you are able to meditate fully. An ashram life is a stepping stone, and eventually you will have to face your life and karma once again in the world.

We all have a divine purpose, and you have to make the whole world your ashram with the faith that your Guru and god are watching and protecting you. You have to go and spread your knowledge and love; the world needs that right now. Some people may stay and live in the ashram for their entire life. This includes those who want to be a monk and send distant prayers and healing to the world, and those who want to avoid the world for a while because they are just not ready to leave yet. The Guru smiles—in his world,

He loves and cares for us all, and we are one in his eyes, but he also puts obstacles in our way so that we can learn from them.

"Ashram is the place where you find men and women of every walk of life, from all branches of Jewish, Christian, Hindu and Muslim religions, Buddhist, Theist, Atheist and Agnostic. Although the United Nations exists for the unity of mankind, still it cannot unite our hearts. Unity that is the ashram's job."

— Shri Brahmananda Sarasvati —

When there's no more hope

And the world seems so unkind

And tears are flowing from my eyes

I turn to you, I run to you

I turn to you, I call out your name.

Are you there? Are you still there?

Are you watching from the blue sky

When I call out your name?

SHRI RAM, MERE RAM.

— Krishna Devi —

Sometimes a Guru sends you out into the world and sometimes he wants you to stay because you need more training and self-realization. If he is honest and if we love him, we surrender to him; he represents godliness in a human form. The meaning of Guru is spiritual master, teacher, and god realized. "Gu" means "darkness" and "ru" means "removes," so a Guru is one who removes darkness.

The relationship between Guru and disciple is the highest love. It is not an earthly love, but instead it is godly, divine love—the real Bhakti yoga. A Guru's love of his disciples is infinite and he takes and dissolves karmas and removes your ego. Sometimes it is not so easy, but once you look into the Guru's eyes, there is no more "you." You disappear into the ocean of love that lasts a lifetime, or even many lifetimes, and that love transforms you and brings you to a higher consciousness and awareness. If you have a Guru in this lifetime, you should feel very lucky because that doesn't happen in every lifetime.

Let me walk on that road that you have passed

Let me sing my song to you alone

Let me whisper your name wherever you go

Just to feel you in the silence.

You never cared for any happiness

Free from fear, free from sadness

Unattached, desireless

Still, you gave your love to all.

— Krishna Devi —

SHRI BRAHMANANDA SARASVATI
(RAMAMURTI S. MISHRA)

Shri Brahmananda Sarasvati is my most beautiful Guru and all of my love flows towards him, with his orange-colored robe and shawl on his shoulder, black stick in his hand, and his eyes like the sun, burning all karmas. He taught me so much and even in his passing and leaving of his body, we still feel his presence in a very real way.

Shri Brahmananda Sarasvati was a great Sanskrit teacher and a real Guru that one can only dream about. He taught the Sanskrit language by chanting, calling it the science of vibration, mostly for the healing of our minds. He gave his life to teaching about the "I-Am," self-awareness and enlightenment, and wrote many stories on the subject. He was constantly chanting the Sanskrit alphabet, verb endings, mantras, sutras, and Kirtan.

He believed that Sanskrit chanting makes one's being divine, dissolves karmas and pain, and purifies the mind, bringing harmony to the senses and to the inner mind. We think that all of these great saints are living in India, meditating in the caves, but I am so happy and feel lucky that this great guru came to America, opened an ashram, and gave his whole being to teach us and open our eyes to a higher consciousness.

When I first came to Ananda Ashram, I arrived with a guitar on my shoulder, carrying a small bag. After I entered the gate, the first person I saw in the doorway of the main house was Guruji. I didn't know that he was the guru, but right away, he put his hand on my head and he said to me,

"Welcome home". I looked into his eyes and I was never the same again.

He had just come out from the sun meditation, so his eyes were like black coal—they were burning. From that day on, he often asked me to sing in part of his program and I wrote many songs about my devotion to Shri Ram, but he always wanted me to play "Hare Krishna Hare Krishna Krishna Krishna Hare Hare, Hare Rama Hare Rama Rama Rama Hare Hare."

One time, I traveled with him and other friends to Syracuse, NY, where he was giving a meditation program. From our ashram, it is a three or four-hour ride by car. When we began the drive, he told me to chant and from that moment on, I was lost in time. I chanted all the way and when we got there, I thought that I had been chanting only twenty minutes. Time just disappeared and I only felt happiness.

JAYA GURU DEVA JAYA, JAYA GURU DEVA

JAYA GURU DEVA JAYA, JAYA GURU DEVA

TASMAI SHRI GURAVE NAMAH

'SALUTATION TO THE GURU'

BABA BHAGAVANDAS

Baba Bhagavandas is the Guru of our Guru. In our ashram, the temple was dedicated for him—the cosmic temple, a magical place. There, you can feel the presence and love of Bhagavandas.

Bhagavandas lived over 150 years and ate very little. He looked very young, not more than forty years old. He was a very magical being and there are stories of his magical ways, his appearing or disappearing. He loved music and chanting and on his birthday, great musicians would come to his tiny place in Bombay and sing and chant for days—this practice still continues today.

SHRI KRISHNA GOVINDA HARE MURARE

HE NATHA NARAYANA VASUDEVA

Most of the great Kirtan leaders have a guru and there is a great love between them. They also believe that after the guru leaves his body, he still guides them. There are many gurus we've had in the past who brought us to higher consciousness. A few that have come to the West are Vivekananda, Krishnamurti, Osho, Satchidananda, Muktananda, Chidananda, Shri Brahmananda, Baba Haridas, Swami Rama, Ramdas, Karunamayi, Amma, and Swami Dayananda. There are many more to come.

It is said that there are many gurus who never left India in physical form, but still traveled in their spiritual form. These include Baba Bhagavandas, Ramakrishna, Sai Baba, Neem Karoli Baba, Babaji, Shivananda, and Shri Nisargadatta

Chapter 10

THE WORLD AND THE YUGAS

We see that this world is full of violence, wars of all kind, depression, racial hate, threats of nuclear and biological war, and global terrorism. Even with all of this, we still dream and hope for peace and harmony.

We are tired of war, violence, racial, religious, and national division; we are crying out to heal the wounds of this earth and bring unity and non-violence. The healing starts in every person's own mind—to be like Saint Francis of Assisi, seeing god in everything. He was a Bhakti Yogi.

—Peace Prayer of Saint Francis—

Lord, make me an instrument of your peace;

Where there is hatred,

Let me sow love;

Where there is injury, pardon;

Where there is doubt, faith;

Where there is despair, hope;

Where there is darkness, light; and

Where there is sadness, joy.

Grant that I may not so much seek

To be consoled as to console;

To be understood,

As to understand,

To be loved as to love;

For it is in giving

That we receive,

It is in pardoning

That we are pardoned,

And it is in dying

That we are born to eternal life.

We are now in the most negative yuga, Kali Yuga, which is full of chaos, problems, war, and sickness. This is the time to chant, in order to heal and save the mind and the world.

They say that with the death of Krishna, Kali Yuga began. When Krishna (Vishnu) incarnates in the future as Kalki, then Kali Yuga ends. He is the final, tenth incarnation of Vishnu, he is the destroyer of darkness, he is tomorrow's incarnation, he is riding on a white horse with wings, he holds a sword in his right hand to destroy Kali Yuga and renew righteousness

In Kali Yuga, our weapon is San Kirtana, chanting god's names. It reverses Kali Yuga.

Kalki does not come to teach, he comes to cleanse this planet and once again establish righteousness on earth for his devotees. He then returns to his eternal abode, leaving the earth again in Satya Yuga:

1st—Satya Yuga: golden age, purity, humans are like gods

2nd—Treta Yuga: silver age, spirituality decreases

3rd—Dvapara Yuga: copper age, negativity is at 50%

4th—Kali Yuga: iron or dark age, negativity and suffering, terrorist acts, hurricanes, tsunamis, etc.

Chapter 11

SOUND OF AUM (OM), MUSIC, AND KUNDALINI

OM NAMAH SHIVAYA GURAVE

NADA-BINDU-KALATMANE,

NIRANJANA-PADAM YATI

NITYAM YATRA PARAYANAH

Salutation to the Nadam, which is the inner guide

And the inner life, the dispenser of happiness to all!

It is the inner Guru appearing as nada, bindu, and kala.

One who is devoted to the inner Guru, the Nada, the

Inner music, obtains the highest bliss.

(Translation by Shri Brahmananda Sarasvati,

From Hatha Yoga Pradipika)

Aum-Om-Pranava Mantra—Anahata Nada—is the voice of silence and the music of nature. This music is everywhere, all of the time. All things are made up of vibration, pulsation, and energy. The unstruck sound is the sound of primal energy; it is a primordial sound and references the creation of the universe, the "Big Bang." These are the original sounds that contain all other sounds—all words, all languages, and all mantras.

God's voice is Aum—the cosmic vibration, a mystical and sacred sound. This is the sound that yogis are listening to in their meditation. It is called Anahata Nada. It was present before creation, when the created universe did not exist. The universe of energy was vibrating in the form of Nada or in the form of divine music, also called the music of the spheres.

" Without inner music, outer music makes no sense. Those musicians who have inner music and at the same time play outer music, they are heavenly musicians, they have the ability to transform the whole world into heaven by their music, and vice versa, those musicians who have no contact with their inner music and play only outer music, they can make anybody crazy by their music."

— Shri Brahmananda Sarasvati —

Heavenly musicians are called Gandharvas. Musical instruments were used by many Indian gods and goddesses: Sarasvati and Sage Narada hold the veena, Shankara plays the damaru and drums, Vishnu holds the conch shell, and Krishna plays the flute.

Man imitates the cosmic sounds and the sounds of environment.
There are two forms of music, the inner and the outer. With meditation on the inner sound, man is freed from the bondage of body and mind. This sound energy will transform you.

Brahma, the creator, conceived music and lord Shiva learned from him; he then passed it to Sarasvati and she passed it to Narada. The developments of notes were created in the Vedic period . Primitive tribes used to sing in one high note, chanting sacred hymns. Later, this developed into two notes, one high and one low, as they sang poetic stories. After that, they sang three main notes, which eventually developed into seven notes.

The Vedic period was very special. Singing, dancing, and playing instruments (veena, flute, mrdanga, damaru) was done in strict rhythm.

As Kirtan moved to the West, more Western melodies were incorporated, using both major and minor scales and different keys—in Indian music, usually only the C Sharp or D notes are used. Also, other instruments were added in the West, like guitar, bass, cello, and violin. Instead of singing in different rag forms, Kirtan developed with a Western scale, in different keys.

In the Vedas, Sama Veda is devoted to the art of music. There are two main schools in Indian music—Hindustani music and Karnatic music, which relate to the North and south of India.

What I enjoy mostly is listening everyday to Holosync recordings from Bill Harris, it is alpha, beta, theta sound vibrations.
These sound waves bring one's mind to a more peacfeul and enlightened state.
Also, Acharya Roop Verma's magical sitar music can bring you into the theta wave state.

When you chant, you also need to know about the mysterious powers of kundalini energy and chakras, and how to awaken each chakra with chanting. Sound is the medicine of the future; through chanting, we become a healer.

The Nadis (energy lines through the body) are like astral tubes carrying prana. Shakti, in the form of serpent energy, is coiled in the base of our spine. The divine mother-energy is hidden in all beings and through chanting and meditation, the Shakti wakes, making a hissing sound, and moves upwards through the spine to each chakra, to ultimately unite us with Shiva.

Chakras in the body are also related to sound vibration. You have to chant some of the Bija Mantras to open and heal the chakras. Chakra means "wheel of light"—they are channels through which spiritual energy flows and manifests in a physical way, moving in and out of our aura. With this, we can awaken our spiritual energy or Shakti.

When the chakra is whirling, it is open, bright, and clear. When it is blocked, the physical and emotional body is then blocked and damaged. At that time fear and desire are found in our chakras. Through correct chanting, we can cause the chakras to turn and whirl.

Muladhara Chakra (LAM)

Location: Root

Element: Earth (name and fame, pleasure, wealth)

Governs: Physical existence and health

Colors: Red, black, brown, grey

Stone: Garnet, onyx, red jasper

God: Ganesha

Goddess: Dakini

Svadhisthana Chakra (VAM)

Location: Below the navel

Element: Water

Governs: Creativity and reproduction

Color: Orange

Stone:Carnelian, orange zincite

God: Narayana

Goddess: Rakini

Manipura Chakra (RAM)

Location:Solar plexus

Element: Fire

Governs: Will and desire

Color: Yellow

Stone: Citrine, yellow sapphire, topa

God :Vishnu

Goddess: Lakini

Anahata Chakra (YAM)

Location: Heart

Element: Air

Governs: Emotion and human love

Color: Green and pink.

Stone:Rose quartz, green tourmalin

Goddess: Kakini

Vishuddhi Chakra: (HAM)

Location: Throat

Element: Ether

Governs: Communication

Color: Blue

Stone: Turqouise, blue lace agate

Goddess: Shakini

Ajna Chakra (AUM)

Location: Third eye

Governs: Bliss, beyond sense of mind

Thought, vision, spiritual love

Color: Dark blue

Stone: Lapis lazulli, sodalite

Goddess: Hakini

Sahasrara Chakra (AUM)

Location: Crown

Ocean of Shiva Shakti

Highest self of divine

Umbilical cord to god

Color: Purple, clear, white

Stone: Amethyst, clear quartz

God: Shiva

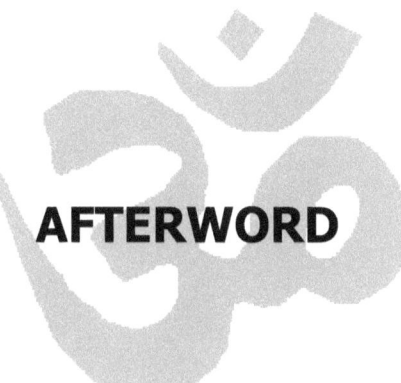

AFTERWORD

You do not have to know or believe all of the things that I wrote, as long as you develop an idea and feeling about them. You just have to chant from your heart with feeling.

We are all spiritual beings having a physical experience. There is a divine way to live on earth—you can serve and help heal the environment, and especially help to eliminate global warming. If you make your own inside god-like, it travels, projects, and bounces onto other people. Through you, they can also feel some happiness, hope, and love.

There is nothing more enjoyable then entering into the world of spirituality, where you feel the pulsation and the universal breath, where time stands still, where your heart is so open that you experience love everywhere, where you see the one in everyone and everything, where you fly high above the sky where the Sun always shines.

These are the results of Kirtan chanting.

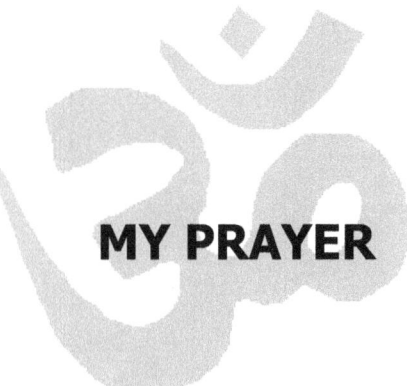

MY PRAYER

MY PRAYER

MAY THE SUN ALWAYS SHINE ON YOU.

MAY THE RAIN WASH AWAY YOUR PAIN AND

SORROW.

MAY ALL THE GODS, RAMA, KRISHNA, SHIVA, JESUS,

MOHAMED, DWELL IN YOUR HEART.

MAY YOUR KIRTAN CHANTING BRING LOVE, BLISS,

DIVINE UNDERSTANDING AND UNITY.

MOST OF ALL, MAY YOU FEEL THE PULSATION, AND

MAGNETIC ENERGY FROM THE CHANTING OF GOD'S

NAME.

OM SHANTIH, SHANTIH, SHANTIH, OM.

— Krishna Devi —

HEALING MANTRAS

MUKHAM KAROTI VACHALAM

PANGUM IANGHAYATE GIRIM

YAT-KRIPA TAM AHAM VANDE

PARAMANANDA-MADHAVAM.

I SALUTE THAT MADHAVA,
THE SOURCE OF SUPREME BLISS,
WHOSE GRACE MAKES THE DUMB ELOQUENT
AND THE CRIPPLE CROSS MOUNTAINS.
(Gita Dhyanam verse 8)

OM SAHA NAVAVATU, SAHA NAU BHUNAKTU,

SAHA VIRYAM KARAVAVAHAI

TEJASVI NAVADHITAM ASTU,

MA VIDVISHAVAHAI.

OM SHANTIH SHANTIH SHANTIH.

May God protect us both in togetherness.
May He nourish us both in togetherness.
May we both work in togetherness with great energy -
physically, mentally and spiritually, individually and
universally,
psychologically and economically, nationally, internationally
and cosmologically.
May our study be vigorous and may our meetings be
effective to strengthen our togetherness in all respect.
May we not hate each other, destroying our togetherness.

— Translated by Shri Brahmananda Sarasvati —

www.ingramcontent.com/pod-product-compliance
Lightning Source LLC
Chambersburg PA
CBHW020245290526
45784CB00003B/1108